The Sleep Advantage

Boost Productivity and Energy with Better Rest

Harmony Royce

DEDICATION

To everyone trying to maintain equilibrium in the face of chaos, and to those who recognize the significant influence that sleep has on our lives. I hope this book serves as a reminder that getting enough sleep is essential, not optional. Let's make relaxation a priority, take care of our health, and realize that we all have boundless potential.

DISCLAIMER

This book contains information that is solely meant to be informative and educational. Although every attempt has been taken to assure the content's correctness and dependability, the author and publisher disclaim all liability for any mistakes, omissions, or results resulting from the use of this information.

Professional medical advice, diagnosis, and treatment cannot be replaced by this book. Please speak with a trained healthcare provider if you have any worries about your health or sleep habits. The information provided should be modified to fit your unique needs and circumstances, as results may differ depending on your situation.

By reading this book, you acknowledge that you use the information at your own risk and that neither the publisher nor the author will be held responsible for any negative effects or losses that may result from using it.

CONTENTS

ACKNOWLEDGMENTS

I would like to sincerely thank everyone who has helped me along the way as I have been writing this book.

I express my gratitude to my family and friends for their constant support and understanding. Even in the difficult times, your confidence in me has been a continual source of inspiration.

A particular thank you to my colleagues and professional mentors who shared their knowledge and ideas on the subject of sleep and productivity. Your advice greatly influenced the breadth and caliber of this effort.

I express my profound gratitude to the researchers, sleep specialists, and medical professionals whose work influenced and informed this book. I am thrilled to be able to share in your incalculable contributions to the field of sleep science.

Finally, thanks to all of the readers, this book would not have been possible without your curiosity and dedication to bettering your health and well-being. I hope the information in these pages will help you change your life and discover the power of better sleep.

Thank you.

CHAPTER 1

COMPREHENDING SLEEP SCIENCE

Sleep is an essential physiological function that is closely related to mental, emotional, and physical health; it is not only a time for rest. This chapter explores the mechanisms, importance, and difficulties of sleep, delving into the interesting science of sleep.

1.1 How the Sleep Cycle Operates

The intricate interaction of brain activity and biological rhythms during the sleep cycle guarantees that the body recovers and continues to operate at its best.

Sleep Stages: An Explanation of NREM and REM

Non-Rapid Eye Movement (NREM) and Rapid Eye Movement (REM) sleep are the two main types of sleep. These phases work together to form a sleep cycle that repeats all night long.

Three sub-stages, each deeper than the previous one, make up the NREM Sleep stage:

Stage 1: The body gets ready for deeper sleep during this light transitional phase. It's over in a few minutes.

Stage 2: A stable sleep phase during which the body temperature decreases, the heart rate slows, and brain activity starts to synchronize.

Stage 3: Also referred to as slow-wave or deep sleep, this is the most restorative stage and is essential for immune system fortification and physical recuperation.

Rapid eye movements, vivid dreams, and increased brain activity similar to awake are the hallmarks of REM sleep. Emotional control and memory processing depend on REM sleep.

Circadian Rhythms' Function

Circadian rhythms, a natural internal clock that is synced with environmental cues like light and darkness, control our sleep-wake cycle. As night falls, the hypothalamus's suprachiasmatic nucleus (SCN) serves as the primary pacemaker, triggering the release of melatonin to encourage sleep. When we feel alert or tired is determined by our circadian rhythms, and disturbances of these rhythms, such as those brought on by shift work or jet lag, can have a significant negative influence on our general health.

The Importance of Regular Sleep Patterns

Irregular sleep schedules disturb the alignment of circadian rhythms with the sleep cycle, resulting in:

- Reduced quality of restorative deep and REM sleep.
- Increased risk of metabolic problems, heart disease, and mental health difficulties. - Impaired cognitive performance and memory consolidation.

Creating regular wake-up and bedtime habits improves the quality of sleep and supports long-term health.

1.2 Sleep-Related Brain and Body Functions

The brain and body are incredibly active during sleep, working on tasks that are critical to preserving general health.

Learning and Memory Consolidation

Sleep is essential for cognitive processes including memory and learning:

- The brain solidifies daytime neuronal connections during REM sleep, assimilating new knowledge into long-term memory.
- NREM sleep, especially slow-wave sleep, reinforces important knowledge while eliminating irrelevant information.
- Better recall of information, abilities, and experiences is made possible by this dual process.

Immune Function and Cellular Repair

Sleep is when the body does a lot of maintenance:

- **Cellular Repair:** Growth hormone promotes bone health, muscle growth, and tissue repair by being secreted mostly during slow-wave sleep.
- **Immune Boost:** Sleep helps the body produce more cytokines and other immune cells, which helps it

fight off inflammation and infections.

Mental Health and Emotional Control

- Processing traumatic or stressful events, lowering anxiety, and enhancing mood stability are all ways that getting enough REM sleep aids in emotional regulation.
- Long-term sleep deprivation has been associated with an increased risk of suicidal thoughts, anxiety disorders, and depression.

1.3 Typical Sleep Issues

Despite the fact that sleep is a normal process, many people suffer from conditions that affect both the quantity and quality of their sleep.

Insomnia: Reasons and Remedies

The inability to fall or stay asleep is the hallmark of Insomnia, which frequently results in daytime irritation and weariness.

- Insomnia can be brought on by stress, worry,

caffeine, erratic schedules, and underlying medical issues.

- Cognitive-behavioral treatment for insomnia (CBT-I) is one behavioral therapy that can help address negative thought patterns and behaviors.

- **Lifestyle Changes:** Symptoms can be considerably alleviated by keeping a regular sleep schedule, cutting back on screen time before bed, and developing a relaxing bedtime ritual.

- **Medications:** Sleep aids may be administered for a brief period of time, but long-term usage is discouraged because of the possibility of dependency.

The illness known as sleep apnea, which is frequently brought on by blockages in the airways (obstructive sleep apnea) or problems with brain signals (central sleep apnea), is characterized by breathing that regularly stops and starts while you sleep.

- One of the warning signs is loud snoring.
- Breathing heavily while you're asleep.
- Oversleeping during the day.

Medications:

- Reducing weight, giving up smoking, and abstaining from drinking before bed are examples of lifestyle modifications.
- **Medical Devices:** Machines that provide continuous positive airway pressure (CPAP) keep airways open.
- **Surgery:** In extreme situations, surgery may be required to realign the jaw or remove blockages.

Restless Leg Syndrome and Other Disturbances

- **Restless leg syndrome (RLS)** is a neurological condition that is typified by an insatiable need to move the legs, usually coupled with discomfort.
- Pregnancy, iron deficiency, and several drugs are triggers.

Management:

- If a verified iron deficiency is found, take supplements.
- Drugs that control dopamine levels.
- Changes in lifestyle, such as avoiding caffeine and exercising frequently.

Effective management of other disturbances, like night

terrors, narcolepsy, and parasomnias, calls for specialized strategies.

Knowing the science behind sleep emphasizes how important it is to our daily existence. We enable ourselves to attain optimal health and vitality by understanding the complex mechanisms of the sleep cycle, acknowledging the crucial roles it plays, and effectively treating abnormalities. After all, the foundation of a good existence is sleep.

CHAPTER 2

SLEEP'S EFFECT ON EFFICIENCY

Sleep is a strong tool that influences physical health, emotional equilibrium, and cognitive abilities in addition to being a biological necessity. Its significant influence on productivity both personal and professional is frequently overlooked. This chapter examines the complex relationship between sleep and productivity, highlighting the advantages it has for cognition, the consequences of sleep deprivation, and its ability to boost output.

2.1 The Advantages of Good Sleep for the Brain

The foundation of the best possible cognitive performance is getting enough good sleep. It has a direct impact on our ability to learn, think, and solve problems.

Enhanced Attention and Decision-Making

- **Attention and Concentration:** Sleep improves the

brain's capacity to sustain focus and attention for extended periods of time. People who get enough sleep are better at setting priorities and removing distractions from their work.

- The prefrontal cortex, the part of the brain in charge of judgment, planning, and decision-making, is strengthened by getting enough sleep. This makes it possible for people to consider their options, foresee outcomes, and come to wise conclusions.

Enhanced Creativity and Problem-Solving

- **Insight Generation:** By forming new connections between concepts that don't seem to be connected, REM sleep in particular promotes creative thinking.

- **Problem Resolution:** Research indicates that people who go to sleep after facing a challenge are more likely to come up with creative solutions than those who remain awake. This phenomena emphasizes how the brain may rearrange and reconstruct data while you sleep.

Easier Information Processing

- **Learning and Memory:** Sleep fortifies brain

networks, allowing the consolidation of newly learned information and abilities throughout the day.

- **Cognitive Efficiency:** Accurate detail recall and effective multitasking are made possible by well-rested brains, which process information more quickly.

Prioritizing good sleep is essential for both personal and professional productivity in today's fast-paced, cognitively demanding world.

2.2 The Price of Lack of Sleep

Lack of sleep has serious consequences for one's long-term health and immediate productivity.

Decreased Performance and Errors at Work

- **Decline in Accuracy:** People who don't get enough sleep are more likely to make mistakes because their judgment and reaction times are slower.
- **Productivity Loss:** Long-term sleep loss reduces productivity since it takes longer and requires more effort to finish tasks.

- **Accidents at Work:** Fatigue dramatically raises the chance of accidents, especially in high-risk occupations like construction, transportation, and healthcare.

Raised Risk of Burnout

- **Emotional Exhaustion:** Sleep deprivation increases stress and impairs resilience, which leaves people more vulnerable to emotional overload.

- **Decreased Job Satisfaction:** Chronic exhaustion lowers motivation and morale by causing emotions of discontent and disengagement.

Long-Term Health Consequences

- **Physical Health:** Heart disease, obesity, diabetes, and decreased immunity are all associated with chronic sleep deprivation.

- **Mental Health:** Long-term sleep deprivation exacerbates mood disorders including anxiety and depression, which further impair wellbeing and productivity.

The cumulative consequences of sleep deprivation

emphasize how crucial it is to make getting enough sleep a top priority.

2.3 Sleep as an Instrument for Productivity

When properly utilized, sleep may be a potent instrument for increasing vitality, improving drive, and developing leadership abilities.

How Sleep Fuels Motivation and Energy

- **Physical Vitality:** Sleep replenishes the brain's capacity for energy by restoring glycogen levels.
- **Mental Stamina:** People with more sleep are more upbeat, flexible, and driven to take on obstacles.
- **Emotional Stability:** Getting enough sleep elevates mood and lowers irritation, which fosters cooperation and teamwork.

Case Studies of Successful People Making Sleep a Priority

Many accomplished people attribute their achievement to making rest a priority:

- **Jeff Bezos:** The Amazon CEO pushes for 8 hours of

sleep weekly, highlighting its importance in keeping sharp decision-making abilities.

- **Arianna Huffington:** After experiencing burnout, the founder of The Huffington Post became a vocal advocate for sleep, underscoring its significance in sustaining creativity and leadership.

- **LeBron James:** The NBA great prefers 8-10 hours of sleep to ensure top athletic and cognitive performance.

These examples indicate that success and sleep are not mutually exclusive; indeed, sleep is a vital enabler of high performance.

The Connection Between Leadership Skills and Sleep

- **Empathy and Emotional Intelligence:** Leaders who get enough sleep are better able to understand people and effectively handle interpersonal situations.

- **Strategic Thinking:** Rested leaders are better at risk assessment, long-term planning, and creativity.

- **Adaptability and Resilience:** Getting enough sleep promotes mental flexibility, which empowers leaders to face uncertainty and setbacks with assurance.

People who understand that sleep is essential to good leadership can use its advantages to motivate and sway others.

Anyone who aspires to brilliance must comprehend how sleep affects productivity. In addition to improving cognitive abilities, getting enough sleep lowers the risk of burnout and exhaustion. People and organizations can achieve greater levels of performance, creativity, and resilience by adopting sleep as a productivity tool.

CHAPTER 3

CREATING THE IDEAL SLEEP ENVIRONMENT

Designing a room that promotes restorative sleep and enhances general well-being is more important than just making it comfortable. From the technology you use to the mattress you select, every aspect of your surroundings affects the quality of your sleep. Let's examine the methods and science involved in creating the ideal sleeping environment.

3.1 Making the Most of Your Bedroom

The cornerstone of your sleeping environment is your bedroom. Observing how it is set up might greatly improve the quality of your sleep.

Selecting the Proper Mattress and Pillows

- **Mattress Selection:** The mattress should satisfy your desired sleeping position and offer sufficient support. For example: A softer mattress that relieves pressure points is better for side sleepers.

- Firmer choices may be preferred by back and stomach sleepers in order to preserve spinal alignment.

- Pillow Aspects to Take into Account: The natural curve of your neck and spine is supported by a quality pillow. Depending on allergies and personal comfort, memory foam, latex, and down are common options.

- To guarantee the best possible support and hygiene, replace your mattress every 7–10 years and your pillows every 1-2 years.

Temperature, Lighting, and Noise Control

- **Temperature:** Research indicates that a bedroom with a lower temperature ideally between 60 and 67°F (15 and 19°C) is better for sleeping. By simulating natural nighttime conditions, cooler temperatures tell the body it's time to sleep.

- **Lighting:** Melatonin, the hormone that induces sleep, is produced more readily in dark environments. To block off outside light sources, use eye masks or blackout curtains.

- **Noise:** Although total quiet is preferable, it's not always feasible. Earplugs or white noise machines can be used to block out distracting noises, such as traffic or loud neighbors.

Decluttering's Effect

- **Psychological Advantages:** A bedroom free of clutter fosters a tranquil atmosphere and lowers stress levels, both of which are beneficial for sleep.

- **Organizational Functions**: Avoid packing nightstands too full, but keep necessities close at hand, such as books or a drink of water.

- **Everyday Tidying:** A calm and sleep-friendly atmosphere can be maintained with a few minutes of daily tidying.

By making the most of these components, your bedroom becomes a haven that promotes restful, deep sleep.

3.2 Technology's Role

Although technology can interfere with sleep, when

utilized carefully, it can also be used to enhance it.

The Science of Blue Light

Blue Light and Screen Time:

- **Managing Exposure:** Blue light from electronic devices inhibits the generation of melatonin and postpones the onset of sleep.

Workable Solutions:

- Steer clear of screens at least an hour before going to bed.
- Make use of blue light-blocking eyewear or put electronics in night mode.
- Choose screen-free relaxation techniques like journaling or reading.

Are Sleep Tracking Devices Beneficial?

- **Wearables and Apps:** Trackers such as fitness trackers keep tabs on sleep habits, offering information on how long and how well people sleep.
- **Benefits:** These tools assist in identifying problems such as irregular schedules or inadequate REM sleep.

- **Limitations:** Orthosomnia, or worry related to sleep, can be brought on by an excessive dependence on trackers. Don't use them as rules; use them as guidelines.

Smart Home Solutions for Better Sleep

- **Automated Lighting:** Smart bulbs may mimic sunrise to promote natural awakening or gradually fade to indicate bedtime.
- **Climate Control:** Smart thermostats keep the temperature in the bedroom at the perfect level all night long.
- **Voice Assistants:** You may use voice commands to control sleep-friendly features or play soothing music on devices like Google Home or Amazon Alexa.

Technology can help improve sleep rather than hinder it if it is used carefully.

3.3 Creating a Relaxing Atmosphere

The environment of your bedroom plays a critical role in

signaling to your body and mind that it's time to wind down.

Aromatherapy and Calming Scents

- **Essential Oils:** Scents including lavender, chamomile, and sandalwood have been demonstrated to induce relaxation and reduce anxiety.

- **Delivery Techniques:** To add relaxing scents to your bedroom, use scented candles, pillow sprays, or a diffuser.

- **Consistency:** Establish a routine that signals your brain to unwind by associating a specific fragrance with going to bed.

Sound Machines and White Noise

- **White Noise:** These devices create steady sound frequencies that drown out distracting sounds, allowing you to sleep for longer periods of time.

- The sounds of nature, such as rain, waves in the ocean, or the atmosphere of a forest, offer a tranquil setting for slumber.

- **Personalization:** Try out various sound

configurations to see what suits you best.

Customizing the Area for Comfort

- **Textures and Fabrics:** For maximum comfort, spend money on premium bedding materials like bamboo or breathable cotton.
- **Colors:** Choose soothing colors that inspire peace, such as blues, greens, or neutrals.
- **Decor:** Showcase simple yet significant objects, such as framed pictures or a beloved work of art, to evoke coziness without overpowering the senses.

Creating a calm environment in your bedroom makes it feel like a haven, which facilitates winding down and getting ready for a good night's sleep.

By carefully planning your sleeping space, you can establish circumstances that promote both the amount and caliber of sleep. A well-designed bedroom, thoughtful technology use, and a calm environment all contribute to better sleep, which in turn improves your general well-being and productivity.

CHAPTER 4

CREATING A SLEEP-ENHANCING ROUTINE

One of the best strategies to enhance the quality of your sleep is to create a regular and deliberate sleep schedule. A well-designed routine lowers stress, improves general well being, and gets your body and mind ready for sleep. Let's examine how developing a sleep-enhancing habit can be facilitated by stress reduction, mindful eating, and pre-bedtime rituals.

4.1 Rituals Before Bedtime

In order to tell your brain that it's time to go from the active demands of the day to the restorative stage of sleep, pre-bedtime routines are essential.

The Value of Winding Down

- **The Viewpoint of Biology:** The body needs time to transition from wakefulness to sleep; it doesn't shut

23

off all at once. The parasympathetic nervous system, which lowers heart rate and encourages relaxation, controls this process.

- **Applications in Practice:** To facilitate your body's natural shift, dedicate 30 to 60 minutes before bed to relaxing activities. Steer clear of emotionally taxing conversations, work-related activities, and strenuous exercise.

Stretching and Meditation as Relaxation Techniques

Meditation:

- Deep breathing techniques and mindfulness meditation lower cortisol levels, which eases mental stress.

- Calm and Headspace are apps that offer regular routines to help calm the mind, as are guided meditations.

- Stretching gently relieves the physical stress that has built up throughout the day.

- Concentrate on postures that promote circulation and muscle relaxation, such as child's pose, forward folds, and seated twists.

The Significance of Light Activities and Reading

- **Reading:** To soothe the mind without causing worry or excitement, use non-stimulating stuff like fiction or motivational tales.

Light Activities:

- Take part in pastimes like puzzle solving, knitting, or drawing.
- Steer clear of screen-based activities to limit your exposure to blue light, which can inhibit the creation of melatonin.

You may establish a consistent routine that promotes sound sleep by introducing relaxing rituals into your pre-bedtime routine.

4.2 Taking Care of Everyday Stress

One of the biggest obstacles to getting a good night's sleep is stress. Learning efficient stress-reduction techniques will greatly enhance your capacity to relax at night.

Stress-Reduction Techniques for Improved Sleep

- **Mindfulness Exercises:** Techniques such as progressive muscle relaxation or yoga aid in the release of physical tension and foster serenity.
- **Time management:** To lessen stress at the end of the day, arrange your chores using strategies like the Pomodoro method or prioritization.

Gratitude Practices and Journaling

Journaling:

- Putting your problems in writing before bed will help you process and put them aside for the evening.
- To feel more in control and less anxious, make a list of the things you need to do the following day in your journal.

Gratitude Practices:

- By thinking back on three good things that happened to you that day, you can divert your attention from problems.
- Better sleep and mental wellness have been associated with this practice.

Balancing Work-Life Demands

- **Set Boundaries:** To avoid work obligations

interfering with your leisure time, set clear deadlines.

- Make leisure a priority by setting aside time for enjoyable pursuits like hobbies, family time, or taking walks in the outdoors.

Your body and mind will be more ready for sleep if you can effectively manage your stress.

4.3 Nutrition and Hydration

The foods you eat during the day, especially right before bed, have a big influence on how well you sleep.

Foods That Encourage or Inhibit Sleep

Foods That Encourage Sleep

- **Bananas:** Packed with potassium and magnesium, they aid in muscular relaxation.
- Magnesium, which is present in almonds, promotes sound sleep habits.
- **Cherries:** A melatonin-producing natural food.

Foods That Hinder Sleep:

- Acidic or spicy foods might induce indigestion, which can interfere with sleep.
- Blood sugar surges from sugary snacks can make it more difficult to fall asleep.

Caffeine and Alcohol: Timing and Impact

Caffeine:

- Steer clear of coffee, tea, or energy drinks in the afternoon or evening as caffeine remains in your system for 6 to 8 hours.
- Nearer to bedtime, choose herbal teas like valerian root or chamomile.

Drinking alcohol:

- Although drinking alcohol can make you feel drowsy at first, it interferes with REM sleep and can cause awakenings at night. Avoid and limit drinking between two and three hours before bed.

Hydration Strategies

Hydration Without Late-Night Interruptions:

- Drink plenty of water during the day to avoid being

very thirsty at night.

- Cut back on fluids one to two hours before bed to reduce the frequency of midnight potty breaks.

A balanced internal environment is supported by mindful eating and drinking practices, which establish the prerequisites for restful sleep.

You can develop a sleep-enhancing regimen that encourages relaxation, lowers stress levels, and maximizes your body's capacity for rest and recuperation by incorporating these techniques into your everyday life. A methodical approach to stress reduction, diet, and pre-bedtime routines guarantees that your days are fruitful and your evenings are rejuvenating.

CHAPTER 5

The Role of Physical Activity in Sleep

Exercise is essential for enhancing general health and the quality of sleep. Frequent movement, whether it be through outdoor activities, mild yoga, or structured exercise, helps your body get ready for a good night's sleep, lowers stress levels, and regulates your circadian rhythms. This chapter explores the ways in which various types of physical activity affect sleep and offers practical tips for incorporating them into your daily schedule.

5.1 Workout to Improve Your Sleep

Although the advantages of exercise vary depending on the type, time, and intensity, it is a potent tool for improving the quality of sleep.

Optimal Times for Exercise

Morning Exercise:

- Your circadian rhythms are strengthened and you feel more alert throughout the day when you exercise in the morning because it exposes your body to natural light.

- Exercise in the morning has been linked to deeper, more restful sleep at night, according to studies.

- Exercise for the Afternoon: - Body temperature is raised by physical exertion in the late afternoon or early evening. Later, when it cools down, it tells the body it's time to go to sleep.

Evening Exercise

- High-intensity workouts near bedtime can raise adrenaline and make it more difficult to fall asleep, but moderate evening workouts might not have a negative impact on everyone.

Sleep Enhancing Exercise Types

Cardiovascular Activities

- Swimming, cycling, and running increase heart rate and enhance general fitness, which is associated with improved sleep patterns.

Strength Training:

- Resistance training enhances deep sleep and lowers anxiety.

- Include exercises involving bodyweight or weightlifting multiple times each week.

- Walking, tai chi, and dancing are examples of low-impact activities that encourage relaxation without putting undue strain on the body.

Avoiding Overtraining and Its Effects

The Dangers of Overtraining:

- Excessive cortisol levels, chronic exhaustion, and insomnia can result from pushing your body too hard.

- Muscle aches, mood fluctuations, and sleepless nights are some of the symptoms.

Balanced Approach:

- Make sure you take enough days off in between strenuous exercise.

- Make recuperation methods like foam rolling, staying hydrated, and eating a healthy diet a priority.

By matching your workout routine to your body's requirements, you may lay the groundwork for regular, restful sleep.

5.2 Stretching and Yoga

Stretching and yoga combine mental and physical relaxation to provide special sleep advantages.

Sleep-Focused Yoga Routines

Restorative Yoga:

- Stress-relieving and rest-promoting positions that focus on the body.
- Particularly useful poses include the child's position, the legs-up-the-wall, and the reclining bound angle.

Evening Yoga Practices:

- Muscle tension and heart rate can be decreased with a 15–30 minute practice before bed.
- Examine applications or videos on the internet that focus on yoga for sleep.

Calm Stretches for Relaxation

Shoulder and Neck Stretches:

- Decompress after spending hours in front of a screen or at a desk.

Stretches for the Hamstrings and Lower Back:

- Focus on muscles that could feel tense after extended sitting.
- Spinal Twists: These aid in spinal realignment and encourage relaxation.

Washing Down Breathing Techniques

4-7-8 Breathing:

- Take a 4-second breath, hold it for 7 seconds, and then release it for 8 seconds. This technique lowers stress and relaxes the neurological system.
- **Diaphragmatic Breathing:** To reduce the heart rate and boost oxygen flow, breathe deeply into the diaphragm.

A comprehensive strategy for relaxing the mind and getting the body ready for sleep is to include yoga and stretching in your evening routine.

5.3 Sunlight and Outdoor Activities

In addition to improving mood, being outside is essential for controlling sleep cycles.

The Relationship Between Sunlight and Circadian Rhythms

The Effect of Sunlight:
- Natural light has a crucial role in regulating the circadian rhythm. It aids in the production of melatonin, a hormone that is necessary for sleep.
- Getting 20 to 30 minutes of sunshine in the morning helps to correct your internal clock and encourage alertness throughout the day.

Evening Light Avoidance:
- To promote the generation of melatonin naturally, reduce exposure to artificial blue light after sunset.

The Calming Effects of Nature Walks

Advantages of Walking in Nature

- Walking in green areas lowers cortisol levels, elevates mood, and promotes better sleep.
- Hiking and beach walks are examples of activities that mix mental relaxation with light activity.
- Walking barefoot on grass or sand can improve emotions of serenity and a sense of connectedness to the natural world.

Including Outdoor Time in Your Daily Routine

Lunchtime Walks:

- To improve your mood and catch some sunshine, take a short stroll during breaks.

Weekend Activities:

- To keep active and in touch with nature, organize outdoor pursuits like picnics, gardening, or group treks.

A quick and easy method to align your sleep schedule with the natural world is to spend time outside.

A key component of proper sleep hygiene is incorporating exercise into your daily schedule. Movement, whether it be through mild yoga, organized exercise, or time spent outside, not only enhances physical health but also gets your body and mind ready for deep, restful sleep. You can use physical activity to improve the quality of your sleep and your general well-being by customizing your activities to fit your preferences and lifestyle.

CHAPTER 6

Developing Your Power Nap Skills

Power naps are a frequently underappreciated strategy for improving cognitive function, regulating fatigue, and increasing productivity. A quick nap is an essential component of a comprehensive sleep plan since, when done properly, it may revitalize the body and the mind. This chapter addresses when naps might not be the best course of action, provides best practices for productive naps, and examines the benefits of napping that have been supported by science.

6.1 Advantages of Sleeping

More than just a midday treat, napping has been shown to be a scientifically supported way to rejuvenate and enhance both mental and physical function.

Improving Memory and Alertness

Enhanced Cognitive Function:

- A well-timed nap can enhance reaction times, strengthen attention, and make you more alert for hours afterward.

- According to research, short-term alertness gains from a 20–30 minute nap can be comparable to those from a full night's sleep.

Memory Consolidation:

- Light NREM sleep, in particular, during naps, helps reinforce knowledge acquired during the day.

- Students, professionals, and anybody else working on learning assignments can particularly benefit from this.

Recovering from Lost Sleep

Mitigating Sleep Debt:

- Naps can help make up for part of the sleep that has been lost when nighttime sleep is insufficient. Those who work shifts or have erratic sleep schedules will find this very useful.

Preventing Sleep Deprivation Effects:

- Momentary naps can mitigate the negative impacts of partial sleep deprivation, including mood fluctuations and impaired focus.

Overcoming Fatigue During the Day

Energy Restoration:

- A brief nap can give you a boost of energy to fight off mid-afternoon fatigue, also known as the "post-lunch dip."

Enhanced Physical Performance:

- By providing muscles and the mind with a little break, naps help athletes and physically active people recover and increase endurance.

When taken properly, naps are a potent remedy for everyday weariness and cognitive deterioration.

6.2 Best Practices for Napping

It's crucial to adhere to a few tried-and-true rules in order to get the most out of naps.

Optimal Sleep Duration

Short Naps (10-20 Minutes):

- These are ideal for increasing energy and alertness without going into deep sleep stages, which might make you feel groggy.

- **Moderate Naps (30-60 Minutes)**: These naps enhance memory retention and decision-making abilities by allowing for both light and deep sleep.

- However, if not taken at the right time, they could cause minor grogginess.

- A complete sleep cycle, which includes REM sleep, can improve emotional fortitude and creativity. This is why long naps (90 minutes) are recommended.

- It is best saved for situations involving severe sleep deprivation.

Timing Naps for Maximum Effect

Mid-Afternoon Sweet Spot:

- In order to take advantage of the natural drop in circadian rhythms, the ideal time to nap is usually between 1:00 PM and 3:00 PM.

- Avoid taking naps too late in the day because this can disrupt your sleep at night.

Think About Your Schedule:

- Adjust your nap time to fit your daily needs, making sure you have enough time to wake up completely before starting important duties.

Prevent Post-Nap Fatigue

Reduce Sleep Inertia:

- The sense of drowsiness or confusion that follows a deep sleep is known as sleep inertia.
- Napping for less than 30 minutes keeps the body from going into deeper sleep stages, which lessens grogginess.

Wake-Up Strategies:

- To rapidly overcome grogginess following a nap, use natural light, exercise, or a glass of water.

Following these guidelines guarantees that naps continue to be a useful tool rather than a cause of interruption.

6.3 When Not to Take a Nap"

Even if taking a nap has many advantages, there are some situations in which it could be more detrimental than beneficial.

Indications That Napping Interrupts Sleep at Night

Difficulty Falling Asleep at Night:

- If taking naps makes you feel too awake at night, it may be an indication that you should cut back on how often or how long you take them.
- Those who experience insomnia or poor sleep quality may discover that taking naps makes their problems worse. This is known as fragmented sleep patterns.

Alternatives to Napping

Engaging Activities:

- To improve alertness, substitute a quick walk or some stretching for a nap.

Mindfulness Practices:

- Deep breathing techniques or meditation can boost vitality and relaxation without endangering sleep.

Nutritional Boosts:

- To maintain energy levels, choose nutritious snacks high in complex carbohydrates and protein.

Overcoming Mid-Day Slumps Naturally

Optimize Your Environment:

- Make sure your workstation is well-organized, has enough lighting, and is kept at a suitable temperature to lessen weariness.

- **Caffeine and Hydration:** To stay alert, drink plenty of water and, if needed, take small doses of caffeine early in the day.

- Your body and mind can be rejuvenated by taking brief pauses that involve movement or exposure to fresh air.

Sometimes it's better to skip a nap, especially if it conflicts with your overall sleep objectives.

Finding the ideal balance between productivity and rest is

key to mastering the power nap. When used carefully, naps can improve physical and mental function, help manage sleep debt, and act as a rapid recharge. Using this tool to assist your general health and productivity requires knowing the advantages, following best practices, and knowing when to avoid naps.

CHAPTER 7

A symbiotic relationship exists between sleep and mental health, with one having a substantial influence on the other. Sleep problems can make mental health issues worse, even if getting enough sleep promotes emotional stability and resilience. This chapter examines the close relationship between sleep and mental health, provides coping mechanisms for anxiety at night, and describes when and how to get professional assistance for sleep and mental health problems.

7.1 The Link Between Mental Health and Sleep

A vital component of mental health, sleep affects mood, thought processes, and emotional control. It is clear why making sleep a priority is crucial for psychological well-being when one understands how sleep and mental health interact.

The Impact of Sleep on Mood Regulation

Emotional Stabilization:

- Getting enough sleep promotes stable, balanced emotional reactions. Anger, impatience, and stress sensitivity can all be exacerbated by little sleep.
- Sleep ensures that the brain processes and recovers from emotional events efficiently, which improves our ability to manage everyday challenges.

Mood Disorders:

- Mood disorders including depression and anxiety are closely associated with sleep deprivation. Frequent sleep deprivation impairs the brain's ability to control emotions.

The Bidirectional Relationship Between Sleep and Anxiety

How Anxiety Affects Sleep:

- Anxiety frequently causes hyperarousal and overthinking at night, which delays the start of sleep and lowers the quality of sleep.

How Sleep Affects Anxiety:

- Lack of sleep causes the brain's amygdala to become more active, which raises anxiety levels. Conversely, restorative sleep mitigates worry by increasing emotional stability.

The Vicious Cycle:

- Poor sleep and anxiety feed into each other, producing a cycle where one exacerbates the other. Breaking this loop is crucial for mental health rehabilitation.

Sleep's Impact on Depression Management

Improving Cognitive Function:

- Sleep supports the prefrontal cortex, responsible for decision-making and focus, typically weakened in depression.

Reducing Symptoms:

- Regular sleep patterns might ease some depressed symptoms, boosting motivation and energy levels.

- The importance of a consistent sleep schedule is emphasized by the fact that sleep management frequently improves the effectiveness of antidepressant therapy.

Sleep plays a fundamental role in mental health, impacting everything from emotional stability to the healing process from severe psychological disorders.

7.2 Getting Rid of Nighttime Nerves

A typical obstacle to getting a good night's sleep is anxiety, which frequently shows itself as sleeplessness, restlessness, and racing thoughts. By putting specific tactics into practice, anxiety at night can be controlled and sleep quality enhanced.

Behavioral-Cognitive Methods

Behavioral-Cognitive Therapy for Sleep Disorders (CBT-I):
- focuses on recognizing and changing harmful ideas and actions that interfere with sleep.
- To combat sleep-related concerns, strategies include cognitive restructuring, sleep restriction, and sensory control.

Reframing Negative Thoughts:

- Train yourself to recognize worrisome thoughts related to sleep and replace them with affirmations that are constructive, like "Resting is beneficial even if I'm not asleep."

Breathing Exercises and Visualization

Deep Breathing:

- Practice diaphragmatic breathing by taking a deep breath through your nose for four counts, holding it for seven, and then slowly exhaling for eight. The nervous system is calmed by this.
- To relieve physical tension, gradually tense and release muscle groups from head to toe using progressive muscle relaxation.
- To help divert attention from distracting ideas, visualize a peaceful setting, like a forest or beach.

Reducing Rumination and Overthinking

Mindfulness Practices:

- Practice mindfulness meditation to stay in the

moment and lessen the propensity to ruminate about the past or the future.

The Worry Journal:

- To "offload" worries before bed, write down apprehensive thoughts earlier in the evening.

Setting Boundaries:

- Establish a "no-problem-solving" rule before bed to prevent overthinking and promote mental relaxation.

Using useful strategies to deal with anxiety at night might help end the worry cycle and create space for healthy sleep.

7.3 Getting Expert Assistance

Sometimes outside assistance is needed to manage sleep and mental health issues. Comprehensive care is ensured by knowing when to seek professional assistance and being aware of your options.

When to See a Sleep Specialist

Chronic Insomnia:

- If you have trouble falling asleep three or more

evenings a week for several months, you may need to see a sleep specialist.

Unusual Sleep Patterns:

- A sleep specialist should be seen for an evaluation of sleep problems such as hypersomnia, sleep apnea, or restless legs syndrome.

- Even with enough sleep, persistent weariness, memory problems, or mood swings could be signs of an underlying sleep disorder.

Insomnia and Anxiety Treatment Options

Cognitive-Behavioral Therapy (CBT):

- CBT treats anxiety and insomnia by teaching people how to control their thoughts, feelings, and actions that disrupt their sleep.

Psychiatric Support:

- Medication and treatment can control neurotransmitter activity, enhancing mood and sleep for people with severe anxiety or depression.

Sleep Hygiene Coaching:

- A counselor or therapist can offer tailored advice on creating and sustaining sound sleeping practices.

Creating a Holistic Mental Health Plan

Integrative Approach:

- Address sleep and mental health issues by combining lifestyle modifications, counseling, and, if necessary, medication.

Regular Monitoring:

- Monitor the development of sleep and emotional well-being using digital tools or journals to evaluate progress over time.

Support Networks:

- Talk to trusted people or support groups to exchange stories and get support.

For people who are having trouble understanding the intricate relationship between sleep and mental health, professional help is a great resource.

Making sleep a priority is essential to preserving and enhancing mental health. People may fully benefit from restorative sleep by realizing the link between sleep and mental health, putting nocturnal anxiety-fighting techniques into practice, and getting help from a professional when needed. By doing this, individuals lay the groundwork for mental clarity, emotional fortitude, and general psychological well-being.

CHAPTER 8

SLEEP DURING VARIOUS LIFE STAGES

As people age, their sleep needs and habits change according to biological, social, and psychological variables. For general wellbeing, it is essential to comprehend how to maximize sleep for various life phases. This chapter explores the distinct sleep requirements of kids, teens, adults, and seniors, providing information and solutions to the problems at each stage.

8.1 Kids and Teenagers

Children's and adolescents' growth and development are fundamentally influenced by sleep. Developing healthy sleep habits in these early years can pave the way for long-term well-being.

Developing Healthy Sleep Habits Early

Regularity is Key:

- Children can more easily fall asleep and wake up naturally when they have regular bedtimes and wake times because they help control the circadian cycle.

Age-Appropriate Sleep Durations:

- School-aged children benefit from 9–12 hours per night, toddlers need 11–14 hours, and infants need 14–17 hours. Teenagers require eight to ten hours, but social and academic pressures frequently cause them to receive less.

- The following are some positive associations with sleep: Establish a relaxing bedtime routine that include reading or listening to relaxing music. Children benefit from this because they learn to identify nighttime with relaxation rather than resistance or tension.

Controlling Screen Time and Bedtime Routines

Restricting Screen Exposure:

- Blue light from screens delays the onset of sleep by inhibiting the production of melatonin. Establish a "screen curfew" that lasts from one to two hours before bed.

Going to Sleep:

- Promote peaceful substitutes for nighttime screen time, such as journaling, sketching, or mindfulness exercises.

Parental Involvement:

- Set an example of excellent sleep hygiene by setting screen time limitations and making sleep a priority for yourself.

Resolving Growth Spurts and Sleep Disruptions

Comprehending Growth Hormone Production:

- Since growth hormone is released during deep sleep, getting enough sleep is crucial for growth.

Managing Sleepwalking and Nightmares:

- After a child experiences a nightmare, reassure them;
- If sleepwalking happens often, see a pediatrician.

Adolescents and Delayed Sleep Phase Syndrome (DSPS):

- Teenagers frequently have a change in their circadian rhythm, which makes them favor later wake and sleep periods. Encourage regular sleep schedules while supporting their biological changes.

When their sleep demands are satisfied, kids and teenagers flourish, promoting physical development, emotional stability, and cognitive development.

8.2 Adults

Adults' sleep patterns are frequently influenced by conflicting demands from their own interests, families, and jobs. Long-term productivity and health depend on adjusting to these difficulties while making rest a priority.

Modifying Sleep Plans to Meet Life's Needs

Comprehending Sleep Cycles:
- Adults need 7-9 hours of sleep every night, usually spread out over 4-6 90-minute sleep cycles. For the best restorative effects, schedule bedtime to coincide with these periods.

Adjusting for Shift Work or Parenting:
- Shift workers should simulate evening by using

white noise and blackout curtains. Young children's parents can share sleep disturbances by taking turns handling evening duties.

Managing Work, Family, and Sleep

The Significance of Time Management:

- Set priorities for your daily responsibilities to prevent them from interfering with your sleep schedule. As much as feasible, assign tasks to others to help them feel less stressed.
- Establish clear boundaries between your personal and professional lives by, for example, refraining from sending work emails after a specific hour.

Making Sleep a Shared Value:

- Promote family-wide sleep schedules to provide everyone the chance to relax and recharge.

The Changing Role of Sleep in Productivity

Quality Over Quantity:

- Pay attention to the quality of your sleep by adopting practices like cutting back on caffeine and sticking to a regular workout schedule.

Napping for Energy:

- During really hard days, quick 20-minute power naps might help you regain focus and alertness.

Sleep as a Competitive Edge:

- Getting enough sleep improves creativity, problem-solving, and decision-making, all of which are critical abilities for both professional and personal development.

Adults can preserve their physical well-being, mental acuity, and emotional equilibrium by recognizing and resolving their particular sleep issues.

8.3 Seniors

As people age, their sleep patterns gradually change, frequently resulting in problems like insomnia, pain, or fragmented sleep. Maintaining health and vigor in older adults requires a focus on sleep quality.

Aging-Related Sleep alterations

Changes in Circadian Rhythm

- As a result of internal clock alterations, seniors frequently have earlier bedtimes and wake-up times. To accommodate these shifts, scheduling should be kept consistent.

Decreased Deep Sleep:

- As people age, they get less deep, restorative sleep. Improve the sleeping environment and nighttime routine as a way to make up for it.

- The prevalence of common sleep disorders, such as sleep apnea and restless legs syndrome, increases with age. For assessment and treatment, speak with a medical expert.

Resolving discomfort and Discomfort at Night

Ergonomic Sleep Solutions:

- To reduce joint and muscle discomfort, get supportive mattresses and adjustable pillows.

Managing Chronic Conditions:

- Sleep disturbances can be caused by conditions such as GERD (gastroesophageal reflux disease) or arthritis. To reduce discomfort, heed physician instructions and use positional sleeping techniques.

Mind-Body Techniques:

- Meditation, tai chi, or gentle yoga help ease mental and physical stress, which will improve sleep.

Remaining Active and Involved Throughout the Day

The Value of Daytime Exercise:

- Frequent exercise helps control circadian rhythms, which guarantees sound sleep at night.

Social Engagement:

- Engaging with friends, family, or community organizations helps people feel less alone and improves their mental health, which in turn improves the quality of their sleep.

Sunlight Exposure:

- By increasing exposure to natural light, spending time outside during the day strengthens the sleep-wake cycle.

By addressing age-specific issues and maintaining proactive habits and health, seniors can greatly enhance the quality of their sleep.

Every stage of life has different sleep needs and difficulties, but everyone needs restorative sleep. People can get optimal sleep and its significant advantages at every stage of life by customizing sleep tactics to the particular requirements of each stage, whether it is establishing habits in childhood, managing obligations in maturity, or adjusting to changes in aging.

CHAPTER 9

GETTING PAST SLEEP ISSUES

Changes in the surroundings, erratic schedules, or personal circumstances can all cause sleep difficulties. These interruptions, which range from jet lag to shift work and the responsibilities of parenthood, frequently impair both the quantity and quality of sleep. In order to ensure that restful and restorative sleep is still possible even in less-than-ideal circumstances, this chapter examines workable solutions for these problems.

9.1 Jet lag and travel

Jet lag can result from time zone changes that interfere with the body's natural clock. This illness frequently presents as exhaustion, sleeplessness, or trouble focusing. Its impacts can be reduced with the right planning and methods.

Adjusting to New Time Zones

Prepare in Advance:

- A few days prior to departure, gradually adjust your sleep schedule to the time zone of your destination. For instance, go to bed earlier if you're going east, and stay up longer if you're flying west.

Set Your Watch Ahead:

- As soon as you get on the aircraft, set your phone or watch to the time of your destination. The transition is made easier by this mental preparation.

Sync with Local Times:

- To aid with your body's quicker adjustment, immediately follow local food and sleep schedules after arriving.

Advice for Improved Sleep During Travel

Trip Comfort

- To establish a sleep-friendly atmosphere during the trip, bring an eye mask, noise-canceling headphones, and a neck pillow.
- Hydrate: Drink plenty of water, but stay away from

too much alcohol and caffeine as these can interfere with sleep.

- **Control Light Exposure:** Use sunglasses or sleep masks during daylight if you need to sleep, and seek bright light exposure during the destination's daytime to adjust your circadian cycle.

Managing Overnight Flights and Hotel Stays

- **Choose Optimal Flight Times:** For long-haul flights, consider schedules that fit with your normal sleep cycles whenever possible.

- **Setup of the Hotel Room:** Make sure your room is cool, dark, and silent. To block distracting noises, use earplugs or white noise applications.

- **De-stress Before Bed:** Use relaxation methods to tell your body it's time to sleep, such as reading, stretching, or meditation.

Jet lag can be considerably decreased by carefully controlling your sleeping environment and light exposure, enabling you to completely enjoy your trip.

9.2 Unusual Schedules and Shift Work

Unusual hours and shift work might disrupt your sleep-wake cycle, resulting in chronic exhaustion and possible health issues. You can lessen these impacts and keep a better rhythm by carefully preparing.

Methods for Non-Traditional Work Hours

- **Anchor Sleep:** Determine the essential sleep times that you can safeguard every day, even if they conflict with the conventional bedtime. The secret is consistency.
- **Plan Ahead:** To prevent interruptions, arrange social events, errands, and other obligations around your protected sleep time.

Night Worker Sleep Hygiene

Establish a Sleep Sanctuary

- Block out daylight and daytime sounds with white noise generators and blackout drapes.
- **Restrict Stimulants:** Steer clear of caffeine and large meals four to six hours prior to your scheduled

bedtime. If necessary, choose light snacks instead.

- **Wind Down After Shifts:** To let your body know when it's time to relax, do something soothing like take a warm shower or practice mindfulness.

Using Light Exposure to Reset Rhythms

Bright Light During Work Hours:

- To maintain alertness and reinforce wakefulness, expose yourself to bright lights while working. It can be beneficial to use specialized light treatment boxes.

- **Regulate Morning Light:** To reduce exposure to sunshine, which might postpone the onset of sleep, use sunglasses on your way home from work.

By using these strategies, shift workers can manage erratic schedules without sacrificing their general health and wellbeing.

9.3 Sleep Disruptions and Parenting

Unusual sleep patterns are sometimes brought on by

parenthood, especially in the early years when infants and toddlers need constant care. Even while sleep disturbances are unavoidable, they can be controlled with cooperation and careful preparation.

Managing Sleep Patterns in Newborns

- **Comprehend Infant Sleep Cycles:** Compared to adults, newborns have shorter sleep cycles and wake up frequently for comfort or to eat. Setting reasonable expectations is aided by accepting this as the norm.

- To lower your baby's risk of SIDS (Sudden Infant Death Syndrome), make sure they sleep on their back on a firm mattress without any unsecured toys or material.

- As they get older, start creating regular nighttime routines, such as feeding, bathing, or singing a lullaby, to indicate when it's time to go to sleep.

Sharing Responsibilities with Partners

- **Divide Night Duties**: Take turns taking care of diaper changes or feedings at night so that each partner may receive plenty of sleep.

- **Plan Sleep Recovery:** Find times during the day or on the weekends when both parents can nap or sleep for longer periods of time.

Parental Napping Strategies

- **Make the Most of Your Baby's Naps:** Take naps when your baby does, particularly in the first few months. Your energy can be restored with even short rests.

- **Make an Effective Plan:** Take shorter (20–30 minute) naps to increase alertness during the day and save longer naps for the evening.

- **Steer clear of overcommitting:** Avoid feeling compelled to finish housework when your infant is napping. Make rest a priority to preserve your health and vitality.

Although being a parent is a difficult job, it is feasible to strike a balance between providing care and getting enough sleep if everyone works together and plans ahead.

Although sleep issues like jet lag, working shifts, and parenting conflicts are inevitable, they don't have to result in long-term weariness or ill health. Regardless of the situation, you can overcome sleep barriers and attain peaceful, restorative sleep by implementing specific tactics.

CHAPTER 10

MONITORING DEVELOPMENT AND MAINTAINING

UNIFORMITY

It takes commitment and consistency to get good sleep. Building habits that support peaceful nights and productive days requires keeping track of your progress and staying motivated. This chapter explores practical methods for tracking, assessing, and maintaining your sleep gains over time.

10.1 Tracking Sleep Behaviors

Understanding trends, seeing disturbances, and modifying your routine with knowledge are all made possible by tracking your sleep. You may learn a lot about the quality of your sleep with the correct methods and resources.

Using Sleep Journals and Apps

- **Sleep Journals:** A sleep diary is an easy-to-use yet

efficient tool to record your bedtime, wake-up time, number of hours of sleep, and any nighttime disruptions.

- Make notes about your activities before bed, your consumption of alcohol or caffeine, your stress levels, and your feelings when you wake up.
- Patterns show up over time, indicating the variables affecting the quality of your sleep.

Technology provides sophisticated tools, such as wearable technology and apps, to track movement, heart rate, and sleep stages.

- Fitbit, Oura Ring, and apps like Sleep Cycle and Pillow are a few examples. These offer thorough data that is frequently shown in reports and graphs that are easy to understand.
- Numerous apps provide useful information, including recommending earlier bedtimes or identifying evenings with higher rates of disruptions.

Identifying Progress and Setbacks

- **Indications of Progress:** Getting to sleep faster,

being asleep longer, and waking up feeling rejuvenated are all signs of progress.

- Positive indicators include a decreased need for alarms and an increase in energy during the day.

Resolving Setbacks: It's common to experience brief interruptions due to illness, stress, or travel. Finding the cause and swiftly resuming healthy practices are crucial.

- Examine your sleep records to identify patterns in any persistent problems, and if necessary, seek advice from a sleep specialist.

Data-Based Routine Adjustment

Customized Modifications:

- Modify the timing of your caffeine intake if evidence consistently indicates restlessness following late-day caffeine consumption.

- Getting up too early on a regular basis could indicate that your sleeping environment is excessively bright or noisy, necessitating the use of white noise machines or blackout curtains.

You may continuously improve your sleeping patterns for long-term success by using tools to track your sleep and actively evaluating the findings.

10.2 Maintaining Inspiration

It takes constant determination to maintain sleep improvements. The process can be made fulfilling and long-lasting by encouraging accountability and acknowledging accomplishments.

Celebrating Little Wins

- **Acknowledge Progress:** Honor accomplishments like maintaining a weekly sleep schedule or waking up feeling energized for several days in a row.
- Use incentives that support your objectives, such as a soothing spa day, new bedding, or a favorite pastime.

Pay Attention to the Benefits: Monitor the effects of better sleep on your general health, happiness, and productivity. Thinking back on these successes helps you see how worthwhile your efforts were.

Accountability Partners and Support Groups

- **Partnering Up:** You can establish mutual accountability by discussing your sleep objectives with a friend, relative, or spouse. For instance, you can both agree to avoid using screens right before bed or to wind down at the same time.

- Frequent check-ins help you stay on course and offer support when things go wrong.

Joining a Community: Local support groups or online forums devoted to sleep enhancement can provide companionship and a shared experience. These groups frequently offer fresh viewpoints and tactics that support you in overcoming obstacles and remaining dedicated.

Considering Productivity Increases

Estimate the Effect:

- Note chores accomplished, creativity levels, and mood swings in your productivity log on the days after getting enough sleep.

- Observing observable advantages encourages

sustained adherence to good practices and emphasizes the value of regular sleep.

Using celebration, accountability, and introspection to motivate yourself guarantees that you will continue to prioritize sleep even when life becomes busy.

10.3 Establishing Durable Habits

Making sleep a top priority, implementing long-lasting adjustments, and adjusting as your needs change are all necessary to establishing lifetime sleep health.

Making Sleep a Priority That Cannot Be Negotiated

Dedication to Rest:

- Consider sleep as a vital aspect of your general well-being, on par with diet and exercise.
- Sleep should be planned like any other important activity, with seven to nine hours each night and no needless interruptions.

Delineating Boundaries:

- Explain to others around you the value of resting without interruption and share your sleep priorities.
- For example, inform coworkers that you will not be answering emails after a specific time, or urge family members to observe quiet times.

Developing Sustainable Lifestyle Shifts

Schedule is Crucial:

- Your body's internal clock is anchored by regular sleep and waking hours, which facilitates natural sleep and wakefulness.
- Develop rest-promoting behaviors, such as regular exercise, cutting back on caffeine, and establishing a relaxing evening routine.

Environment Matters:

- To create the perfect sleeping environment, get a firm mattress and pillows, keep your bedroom cool and dark, and reduce noise.
- Maintain comfort and support by routinely evaluating and improving your sleeping arrangement as necessary.

Reevaluating and Adjusting as Life Changes

Remain Adaptable:

- Your sleep schedule may need to shift as a result of life transitions like new employment, aging, or family obligations.
- Track your sleep to determine when disturbances happen and modify your routine to deal with them.

Continuous Learning:

- Keep up with new developments in sleep science and tools or methods that can improve your regimen.
- Make sure your sleep objectives and tactics are in line with your needs and present situation by reviewing them on a regular basis.

You may stay consistent and enjoy the long-term advantages of restful sleep by making sleep a priority and forming routines that change as your life does.

The basis for long-term sleep health is laid by regularly monitoring progress, maintaining motivation, and forming enduring habits. You may overcome obstacles, acknowledge accomplishments, and guarantee that getting enough sleep continues to be a crucial component of your overall health by adopting a deliberate and flexible strategy.

ABOUT THE AUTHOR

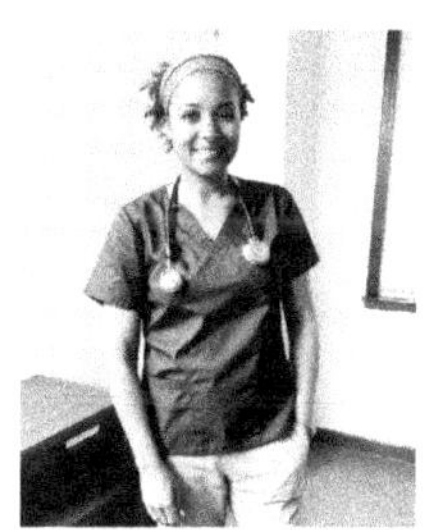 Harmony Royce is a dedicated healthcare worker who has a strong interest in holistic wellness. Harmony's extensive history in various aspects of health and wellness provides her with a wealth of knowledge and expertise that she can utilize in her writing and professional endeavors.

Harmony is a talented author who crafts thought-provoking books that inspire readers to have well-rounded, balanced lives. She writes about a variety of health-related topics, such as diet, exercise, mental health, and mindfulness. Her approachable writing style combines practical guidance with evidence-based research to make complex health concepts approachable and engaging for readers of all ages.

Harmony actively promotes the benefits of holistic health through writing, community workshops, and internet forums. Her mission is to educate and inspire people about the transformative power of self-care and healthy lifestyle choices.

www.ingramcontent.com/pod-product-compliance
Lightning Source LLC
Chambersburg PA
CBHW050819250726
48653CB00006B/2315